INFLUEN

by

DOUGLAS M. BORLAND
M.B., Ch. B. Glass., F.F. Hom.

B. Jain Publishers Pvt. Ltd.
Delhi

Price : Rs. 5.00

Reprint Edition 1998

Published by:
B. Jain Publishers (P) Ltd.
1921, Street No. 10th Chuna Mandi,
Paharganj, New Delhi-110055 (INDIA)

Printed in India by :
J.J. Offset Printers
7, Printing Press Area, Ring Road,
Wazirpur, Delhi

ISBN 81-7021-652-4
BOOK CODE B-2098

Influenzas

By Dr. D. M. Borland

The following lectures on Influenzas are being reprinted by request. They were given by Dr. D. M. Borland at the London Homœopathic Hospital in 1939.

The drugs are not arranged alphabetically, but in the order in which Dr. Borland considered them likely to be of value to the physician and his patients.

GELSEMIUM SEMPERVIRENS

VISUALISE the ordinary, typical influenza case, probably developing over six to eight hours. The patient feels a little out of sorts the day before, possibly a little headachy, a little feverish, has a little indefinite pain, is probably a little catarrhal; he goes to bed, does not sleep awfully well, and next morning feels rotten.

Fortunately, there is a drug in the materia medica which produces exactly that picture, and which will cover a large percentage of the cases of straightforward influenza. The drug is *Gelsemium*. It develops its symptoms fairly slowly and produces exactly the symptom picture given above. Other influenza drugs will be dealt with in due course.

Gelsemium is somewhat slow in onset, and produces primarily a feeling of intense weariness. The patients are very dull and tired, look heavy and are heavy-eyed and sleepy; not wanting to be disturbed but to be left in peace, and yet—the first outstanding symptom—if they have been excited at all, they spend an entirely sleepless night, in spite of their apparently dull, toxic state.

The patient is definitely congested, the face slightly flushed—rather a dull kind of flush—the eyes a little injected, the lips a little dusky; the skin generally is a little dusky, and the surface is definitely moist—hot and sticky.

Another *Gelsemium* symptom is that with the hot, sticky sensation, the patients have a very unstable heat reaction. They feel hot and sticky, and yet have the sensation of little shivers of cold up and down their backs—not actual shivering attacks but small trickles of cold, just as if somebody ran a cold hand, or spilt a little cold water, down their back.

With their general torpor, *Gelsemium* influenza patients always have a certain amount of tremulousness, their hands become unsteady much more quickly than you would expect from the severity of their illness; they are definitely shaky when they lift a cup to try and drink. Frequently linked with the shakiness is a feeling of

1

instability, and very often a sensation of falling. They feel as if they are falling out of bed, particularly when they are half asleep; they wake with a sudden jerk and feel as if they have fallen out of bed.

As one would expect with anyone in this toxic state, the *Gelsemium* patient does not want to make any effort at all; discomforts of every kind are aggravated by moving. With their unstable circulation they are definitely sensitive to cold draughts, which make them shiver.

As a rule, their mouths are intensely dry and the lips very dry; very often dry and cracked, or dry with a certain amount of dried secretion on them. The patients complain of an unpleasant taste, and there is frequently a sensation of burning in the tongue. The tongue itself usually has a yellowish coating—though, sometimes, it is quite red and dry.

Gelsemium influenzas always include a very unpleasant, severe headache. Typically, there is a feeling of intense pain in the occipital region, spreading down into the neck with a sensation of stiffness in the cervical muscles; and, as it is a congestive headache, it is usually throbbing in character.

The patient is most comfortable when keeping perfectly still, propped up with pillows, so that the head is raised without the patient making any effort. With these headaches, the patients often complain of a sensation of dizziness, particularly on any movement.

There is another type of headache sometimes met with in *Gelsemium*. Again, it is congestive in character, but the sensation is much more a feeling of tightness—as if there were a tight band round the head, just above the ears from the occiput right forward to the frontal region. This, also, is very much aggravated by lying with the head low.

Peculiarly, these patients often find relief from their congestive headaches by passing a fairly large quantity of urine.

In nearly all *Gelsemium* influenzas there is a sensation of general aching soreness, an aching soreness in the muscles. This is worth remembering: there are other drugs which have similar pains but are much more deep-seated than the *Gelsemium* pains.

Now for a few details of actual local disturbances.

Most *Gelsemium* patients have that appearance of intense heaviness of the eyelids that is associated with this dull toxic condition. But there is also a good deal of sensitiveness of the eyes themselves, a good deal of congestion, a definite sensitiveness to light, probably a good deal of lachrymation and general congestive engorgement.

There is an apparent contradiction here: despite this occular sensitiveness, occasionally a *Gelsemium* patient becomes scared in the dark and insists on having a light.

These patients get very definite acute coryza, with a fluid, watery discharge, accompanied by very violent sneezing and a feeling of intense fullness and pressure just about the root of the nose. It is not uncommon in *Gelsemium* influenza—where there is this feeling of blockage at the root of the nose—to find a story of epistaxis on forcible clearing of the nose. This, again, is worth remembering, for certain *Mercurius* cases tend to run in the same way.

With their acute coryzas, *Gelsemium* patients, despite a general hot stickiness, very often complain of very cold extremities. (This appears to be a contradiction, and might mislead you when you consider the general heat of the typical *Gelsemium* patient.)

As a rule, in *Gelsemium* influenzas, there is no very marked localised tonsillitis, but much more a generalised, puffy, red, congested throat. There may be a certain amount of enlargement of the tonsils, but it is not the spotty throat that some of the other drugs have.

In spite of the absence of acutely localised symptoms there is often acute pain on swallowing. Swallowing may be actually difficult—with a feeling of constriction or of a lump in the throat—and it is much more difficult when the patients take cold fluids than warm; this is unexpected, considering the dryness of their mouths.

Associated with these conditions of nose and throat, *Gelsemium* influenzas quite frequently have an involvement of the ears. But, in spite of what is recorded in the materia medica, I have not observed the acute stabbing pains that are described under *Gelsemium*; and, where I have tried to clear up such pains with *Gelsemium*, I have not had any success.

Gelsemium is given as one of the drugs that has stabbing pain into the ear on swallowing: in my experience, it has not been effective. *Gelsemium* does get a good deal of roaring in the ears, a feeling of blockage and obstruction and you very often get dullness of hearing, and giddiness; but I have not seen acute earaches respond to *Gelsemium*.

Quite frequently there is an extension downwards, with involvement of the larynx and loss of voice. Associated with the laryngitis, there is liable to be an intensely croupy cough which is almost convulsive in character, coming in spasms and associated with very intense dyspnœa.

Typical *Gelsemium* patients, despite their sweatiness and dryness of mouth, are not usually very thirsty. Occasionally a patient is intensely thirsty, but the typical one is not.

They hardly ever have an appetite—they do not want anything at all. They very often complain of a horrible empty sensation in the region of their chest, often near the heart. This sometimes spreads down into the epigastric region, and they may describe it as an empty feeling; but it is not really a sensation of hunger, and is not associated with any desire for food.

Associated with the digestive system, *Gelsemium* patients often have a definitely yellowish tinge, and actual jaundice may develop. Again, the patient quite frequently develops very definite acute abdominal irritation accompanied by diarrhœa. Usually, the stool is very loose and yellowish but not particularly offensive.

There is quite often a story of intense feeling of weakness in the rectum—an incontinence, or a feeling of prolapse—after the bowels have acted; and there is sometimes a definite prolapse associated with the diarrhœa.

BAPTISIA

BAPTISIA runs very closely to *Gelsemium* in symptomatology. Personally, I look at *Baptisia* as *Gelsemium* exaggerated, more intense.

In contrast to *Gelsemium* patients, *Baptisia* patients are definitely more dusky. They give you the impression that their faces are a little puffy and swollen; their eyes are heavy, but with a congested, besotted look rather than the drooping lids of *Gelsemium*; and lip congestion, present in *Gelsemium*, makes *Baptisia* lips rather blue.

Mentally, *Baptisia* patients are more toxic than *Gelsemium* patients; they are less on the spot; they are confused, finding it difficult to concentrate on what they are doing. They grow a little confused as to the sensation of their body; they may feel that their legs are not quite where they thought they were. Their arms may have definite disturbed sensations: some patients feel their arms are detached and they are trying to re-attach them, others say their arms are numb.

Associated with this is the general *Baptisia* confusion. The patients themselves are not quite clear why they are there, where they are, what they are talking about or trying to discuss; and they are not quite clear whether there is somebody else talking to them, somebody else in the bed. They are simply more fuddled than *Gelsemium* patients.

As you would expect with the slightly more intense toxæmia, all the local conditions are definitely worse. The tongue is definitely dirtier—the typical *Baptisia* tongue is in a pretty foul state. In the early stages it usually has a central coating of yellow, brown or black with a dusky red margin all round.

The patient's breath is always foul. With this very foul mouth, there tends to be a lot of ropy, tough saliva which is apt to dribble out of the corner of the mouth when the patient is half asleep. In consequence, the lips tend to crack and become very foul, and may actually bleed.

Contradictions arise. The *Baptisia* patient is obviously much more ill. He appears to be much more toxic, and more drugged; at the same time he is much more sensitive, with more sensitive arms, legs, back—he is tender all over. He complains of his bed hurting him; any pressure is painful. And, in spite of his toxicity, he is very often restless, constantly on the move, trying to find a comfortable position.

The *Baptisia* patient sweats a lot, but the sweat, in contrast to the somewhat sourish odour of *Gelsemium*, is definitely offensive. This is true of anything in connection with *Baptisia*: it is all offensive. Mouth, breath, sweat, diarrhœa (which *Baptisia* patients incline to) sputum, all are offensive; much more so than one ever finds in *Gelsemium*.

Baptisia mouths and throats, as contrasted with those of *Gelsemium*, are a very much more dusky red—a dusky, dark red. In *Baptisia* there is a strong liability for definite ulcerative conditions to develop about the tonsils and spread up to the soft palate. And again here, strongly noticeable is the accumulation of this filthy, glairy mucus, and the extreme offensiveness.

Occasionally, you find a *Baptisia* throat with fairly extensive ulceration that is strangely insensitive. Commonly, however, the *Baptisia* throat is painful; there is great difficulty and pain on swallowing, a feeling of obstruction, and the swallowing of solids is almost impossible.

As you would expect with this very foul infective condition, there is liable to be an extension into the ears, with a sensation of fullness, obstruction and pain. Very often there is a middle-ear abscess, and not infrequently a tendency to very early development of mastoid infection.

In *Baptisia*, it is much more commonly the right ear and the right mastoid region which is involved. If a mastoid does occur, the prognosis is very serious indeed. Thrombosis occurs very early— and I mean astonishingly quickly—and the prognosis becomes correspondingly worse.

In a *Baptisia* influenza with obvious mastoid developing—tenderness and slight blush over the mastoid region—it is astonishing how

5

the case alters completely within two or three hours of giving *Baptisia*. The patient, from being obviously toxic—so toxic that all the signs of starting meningeal irritation are developing—is equally obviously recovering, as a result of even the first dose of *Baptisia*.

In contrast with *Gelsemium*, *Baptisia* patients are always thirsty. They have a constant desire for water, but if they take much at a time it often produces a sensation of nausea. Taking a little at a time, they are all right, but their thirst is always one of their troublesome features.

Usually, there is not much of a cough in *Baptisia* cases. There is a good deal of dyspnœa, a feeling of oppression in the chest, which is very much worse when they are lying down, and rather better for a current of air; when there is a cough it is usually induced by a sense of irritation in the throat rather than a definite accumulation of sputum in the chest.

In their influenzal attacks, *Baptisia* patients are very liable to have a gastric or liver disturbance. Very often it is associated with acute diarrhœa accompanied by violent tenesmus, a good deal of colic and a bileless stool.

Baptisia patients always have intense aching pains all over. Any part they press is painful and tender; they also have acute pains in their joints, a feeling as if they were sprained or had been bruised; moving is very painful.

BRYONIA ALBA

THE typical *Bryonia* influenza develops, like the *Gelsemium* case, over a period of six to twelve hours. And the appearance of *Bryonia* patients is not unlike that of *Gelsemium* patients. They give the impression of being rather dull, heavy, slightly congested, with a rather puffy face.

Although they are definitely heavy-looking, they do not have the sleepy appearance that you find in *Gelsemium*, nor yet the besotted look of the *Baptisia* patient—something between the two.

Mentally, as stated, *Gelsemium* patients are dull, sleepy, heavy and do not want to be disturbed. *Bryonia* patients are also definitely dull and do not want to be disturbed—but if they are disturbed they are irritable. Irritability is always cropping up in *Bryonia* patients. They do not want to speak, and do not want to be spoken to. They do not want to answer because speaking annoys them, not because they are too tired to do so.

As a rule, *Bryonia* influenzas are very depressed; they are despondent and not a little anxious as to what is happening to them they feel they are ill and are worried about their condition.

6

To their worry about their impending illness they add a very definite anxiety about their business. They talk about it; if they become more toxic, they are apt to dream about it, and it is an underlying thought in the back of their minds throughout their illness.

It is also typical of *Bryonia* influenzas that the patients are difficult to please. They are very liable to ask for something and refuse it when it comes. They want a drink and, when it comes, do not want it. Or, they may ask for a fruit juice drink and, when that comes, say they would much rather have had a drink of plain cold water—they are very difficult to satisfy.

Typically, they have a good deal of generalised, aching pain. They will tell you that it hurts them to move, and yet, very often, *Bryonia* patients are constantly on the move. They are restless and uncomfortable, and move about in spite of the fact that the movement increases their pain.

Get hold of this fact very clearly, because it is so definitely laid down in text-books that *Bryonia* patients are aggravated by motion. Apparently it does hurt them, but they get into this restless state when they will not keep still.

When the patients are restless, find out whether it eases them or not. If it does not, they are probably *Bryonia* cases. If it does ease them, consider one of the other drugs—possibly *Baptisia* or one of the restless drugs, such as *Rhus tox*. It is a point that needs early clarification.

Bryonia patients feel hot, and are uncomfortable in a hot stuffy atmosphere; they like cool air about them. This can be linked with their thirst. They are always thirsty, and their desire is for cold drinks—large quantities of cold water—though, as mentioned above, they may ask for cold, sour things and then refuse them when they are brought.

As a rule, *Bryonia* patients sweat a fair amount, sometimes profusely, with a damp, hot sweat.

Although these patients are sensitive to a hot room, you occasionally find a *Bryonia* influenza with definite rheumatic pains—one or other joint becoming very painful—and who claims that the joint is relieved by hot applications. This is a local contradiction to the general heat aggravation.

There are one or two points which help in differentiation, in connection with local conditions.

There is a very typical *Bryonia* tongue. It is usually a thickly-coated white tongue. The white coating is liable to become dirty in appearance, and may become brown if the disease condition has lasted long, particularly if there is much respiratory embarrassment and the patient is breathing through the mouth.

With that dry tongue, the patients complain, not unexpectedly, of an unpleasant taste in their mouths, very often of a bitter taste, accompanied by fairly intense thirst. As a rule, these patients have rather swollen, puffy, dry lips which tend to crack and may bleed very easily.

In the typical *Bryonia* throat there is the same sensation of extreme dryness, heat and burning. On examination, the tonsillar region and the back of the throat are usually found to be pretty deeply congested; the tonsils are liable to have small, usually white, spots. The throat also is unduly painful on swallowing, which is, of course, the ordinary *Bryonia* aggravation from movement.

All *Bryonia* influenzas have very intense headaches. Usually, the headache is intense, congestive and throbbing; the most common situation for it is in the forehead.

Patients often say they feel as if they have a lump in their foreheads, which is settling right down over their eyes. The pain modality of the headache is that it is very much relieved by pressure— firm pressure against the painful forehead affords great relief to the *Bryonia* headache.

As one would expect, the headache is very much worse from any exertion—talking, stooping or movement of any kind. It is worse if the patient is lying with the head low; the most comfortable position is semi-sitting up in bed, just half-propped up.

Definite neuralgic headaches are found sometimes in *Bryonia* influenzas: general neuralgic pains about the head, with extreme sensitiveness to touch. The whole surface of the scalp seems to be irritated; and it may spread down into the face, on to the malar bones, again with extreme hyperæsthesia.

All *Bryonia* influenzas tend to more or less congestion of the eyes, which may go on to a definite conjunctivitis. The eyeballs themselves are sensitive to pressure; patients sometimes say that it hurts even to screw their eyes up—not an uncommon influenzal symptom.

As a rule, *Bryonia* patients do not have a very profuse nasal discharge. More commonly, they complain of feelings of intense burning and heat in the nose, or of fullness and congestion.

There is liable to be a very early extension of the catarrhal condition into the larynx, with a very irritating, tickling, burning sensation and very definite hoarseness—sometimes actual loss of voice. Also a feeling of rawness, and a very suffocative tight sensation rather lower than the larynx, with a very irritating, bursting, explosive cough.

8

I have not observed much tendency to acute ear involvement in *Bryonia* cases. There is much more a feeling of blockage and stuffing-up of the ears, possibly a certain dullness of hearing, but little more than that.

Bryonia influenzas do not show any very marked tendency to extend into the digestive tract. There are, of course, *Bryonia* abdominal symptoms in other conditions, but I have never seen *Bryonia* indicated in an influenza with definite abdominal symptoms.

There is nearly always troublesome constipation, and a definite lack of appetite which, considering the state of the *Bryonia* mouth, is not surprising. There may be a certain amount of general abdominal discomfort, a feeling of heaviness—almost of solidity—in the epigastrium.

The patients do not want any food and, if pressed to eat, are very often more uncomfortable after it. But as a rule, I have not seen acute gastric disturbances associated with *Bryonia* influenzas. They are much more likely to have a chest disturbance, even a definite pneumonic attack, than a gastric attack.

Of course, if the patient does have a pneumonic attack, it will be the typical *Bryonia* pneumonia, with violent stabbing pains in the chest, a feeling of acute oppression, extreme pain on coughing, pain in the chest on movement with the desire to keep it as still as possible. But this is rather going beyond the uncomplicated influenzas.

EUPATORIUM PERFOLIATUM

THE outstanding point which leads to the consideration of *Eupatorium* is the degree of pain which the patients have. There are very intense pains all over—of an aching character—which seem to involve all the bones of the skeleton, arms, legs, shoulders, back, hips and, particularly, the shin bones.

As a rule, *Eupatorium* influenzas develop rather more quickly than others, and the pains develop very rapidly. The patients say it feels as if the various joints were being dislocated—it is that type of very intense, deep-seated pain. Associated with the pain, there is incessant restlessness; the patients are always moving to try to ease the aching pain in one or other of their bones.

In *Eupatorium* influenzas—a useful differentiation point—the sweat is very scanty. Other drugs which have a very similar degree of bone aching all tend to sweat.

The patients are always depressed. but with a different depression from that of *Bryonia*. They are acutely depressed and definitely complaining; they complain bitterly about the intensity of their pain and, if they are not complaining, they move around in bed, groaning and moaning; and are very sorry for themselves.

In appearance, they usually have a fairly bright flush and a dryish skin, with rather pale lips, in contrast to the deep congested appearance in the other drugs already described. They tend to have a white-coated, thickish fur on the tongue and, instead of the bitter taste of *Bryonia*, they simply have a flat, insipid taste

Eupatorium patients are always chilly; they feel cold and shivery, are sensitive to any draught of air and very often have a sensation of chilliness spreading up the back.

They usually suffer from quite intense headaches. Typically, they complain of extreme soreness of the head, very often most marked in the part that is resting against the pillow.

There is one exception to this: they complain of extreme soreness in the forehead, where there is no pressure at all, and a sensation of pulsation in the occipital region, accompanied by a feeling of intense heat on the top of the head.

They sometimes have a strange surging feeling in the head and, oddly, the surging seems to go from side to side across the top of the head.

Coryza in *Eupatorium* is rather distinctive. The patient has a feeling of intense obstruction—as if the nose is completely stopped-up—and this is accompanied by most fluent discharge with violent and incessant sneezing.

With this coryza there is always marked involvement of the eyes. The margins of the lids look red and inflamed, there is intense lachrymation and a feeling of generalised soreness. They look congested; and there is some degree of photophobia, but not very marked.

Eupatorium patients sometimes develop an extreme hyperæsthesia to smells of any kind. Any odour induces a sense of irritation, aggravates the coryza and, very often, makes them feel sick.

They suffer from an intensely dry throat, which is just generally congested. With it they are very thirsty, with a desire for ice-cold drinks. I remember a *Eupatorium* patient whose one desire was for ice-cream. He did not swallow it but held it in his mouth to cool the burning at the back of his throat.

Care must be taken, however: if *Eupatorium* patients have too much ice water, ice-cream or cold drinks, they are very prone to gastric attacks. Liable to a good deal of eructation of wind anyway; irritation of cold fluids in the stomach may cause a definite bilious vomit.

The catarrhal condition usually avoids the larynx, but the patients complain of intense heat and burning in the trachea. This is accompanied by a very trying cough, which again is accompanied by intense soreness in the chest walls. There are intense aching pains all through the chest muscles, pains which feel as though they are actually in the ribs.

The *Eupatorium* cough is very violent, with scanty sputum, and it seems to hurt the patients from head to toe. It makes their head burst and increases the chest pains, so that they try to restrain the cough or control the chest movement, even while they are coughing, because of the pain. It is a generalised aching pain—as if they were being broken; not the sharp, stabbing pain of *Bryonia*, which is equally as sensitive.

RHUS TOXICODENDRON

THE onset of a *Rhus tox.* influenza is usually gradual and without a very high temperature; it is a slowly progressing feverish attack, which is accompanied by very violent generalised aching.

The aching in *Rhus tox.* is very typical indeed. The patients are extremely restless; their only relief lies in constant movement, constant change of position. If they lie still for any length of time, their muscles feel stiff and painful, and they turn and wriggle about in search of ease. This constant restlessness is the most noticeable thing about *Rhus tox.* patients on first sight.

They are very chilly, and very sensitive to cold. Any draught or cold air will aggravate all their conditions, and is enough to aggravate their coryza and start them sneezing; an arm outside the bedcovers becomes painful and begins to ache, and so on.

Understandably, *Rhus tox.* patients are extremely anxious; they get no peace at all, and are mentally worried, apprehensive and extremely depressed. The depression is not unlike that of *Pulsatilla*; the patients go to pieces and weep.

With all the restlessness and worry, they become very exhausted and, considering that their temperature is quite moderate, unduly tired-out, almost prostrated.

Rhus tox. patients invariably have extremely bad nights. It is very difficult for them to get to sleep because of their constant discomfort; when they do sleep, their sleep is very disturbed, full of all sorts of laborious dreams—either that they are back at work, or making immense physical effort to achieve something.

They sweat profusely. And the sweat has a peculiar sourish odour, the sort of odour one used to associate with a typical case of acute rheumatic fever.

11

These patients always have intensely dry mouths and lips, and very early in their disease they develop a herpetic eruption which starts on the lower lip—small crops of intensely sensitive vesicles that spread to the corners of the mouth. These usually develop within the first twelve hours of their illness.

The typical *Rhus tox.* tongue is very characteristic. It has a bright red tip and a coated root, the coating varying from white to dark brown. Instead of the typical triangular red tip, some patients have a generalised dry, red tongue which tends to crack, is burning hot and very painful.

Associated with the sensitiveness of their lips and tongue, these influenza patients tend to very acute dental neuralgia; their teeth become very sensitive and are painful if touched.

They develop extremely sore throats—dry and burning. On examination, the throats appear to be œdematous. They are very sensitive on swallowing, particularly empty swallowing; and it is easier for them to take solids than fluids.

Rhus tox. patients have very violent attacks of sneezing. They describe them as usually more troublesome at night, and so violent as to make them ache from head to foot. As a rule, the nasal discharge is somewhat greenish in colour.

They get very troublesome tickling irritation behind the upper part of the sternum. This produces a persistent and very racking cough, with which they develop a raw, burning sensation in the larynx, which very often progresses into definite hoarseness.

This hoarseness is very characteristic: the patients complain of a feeling as if their larynx were full of mucus. They feel that they cannot clear their voices until they have coughed the mucus out, and yet the effort of coughing feels as if it is almost tearing or scalding their larynx.

As a rule, there is a good deal of congestion of the eyes—generalised congestion, with very marked photophobia and a good deal of lachrymation.

They suffer from rather severe occipital headaches, with a sensation of stiffness down the back of the neck and, very often, marked giddiness on sitting up or moving. They often complain of a sensation of weight in the head, as if it were an effort to hold it up.

Rhus tox. patients often complain of a feeling of intense heat inside, and yet their skin surface feels the cold. They are sweating profusely and any draught seems to chill them—they feel the cold on the surface—but they feel burning inside.

In these influenzas, the patients are very apt to have violent attacks of nodular urticaria, scattered anywhere over the body and intensely irritable.

12

The patients are not usually markedly thirsty, though they do like sips of water to moisten their very dry mouths and throats.

I have seen a *Rhus tox*. influenza go on to a definite enteritis with violent abdominal pain; pain down in the right side, down in the cæcal region, with extreme restlessness, tenderness and very stinking diarrhœa.

But I have seen only the one case. It responded very well to *Rhus tox*. There was the typical tongue and general anxiety and restlessness, general aching pain, sweating and chilliness; and it was more on the general than on the local abdominal symptoms that I prescribed *Rhus tox*.

PYROGENIUM

PYROGENIUM influenza patients usually run a fairly high temperature. Typically, they are flushed, hot, sweaty and somewhat congested-looking. They very often complain of a sensation of burning heat, and feel horribly oppressed by it.

Most of the *Pyrogenium* influenza patients that I have seen have been over-active mentally. They tend to be very loquacious and chatter away readily, and become definitely excited in the evening maybe even delirious.

They are very much troubled with sleeplessness, due again to excessive mental activity; if they become toxic, they may get a slight degree of delirium with a sensation of uncertainty as to where they are. They quite frequently wake up bright and clear and describe unpleasant dreams of having to try and collect themselves from all over the bed—but that is more in their sleep than when they are awake.

A constant *Pyrogenium* indication is that, though the patients feel so very hot and uncomfortable, they are sensitive to any draught. It makes them shiver at once—very much as in *Mercurius*—and they quite frequently get little shivers, almost little rigors, intermingled with their feeling of intense heat. Very often the patient feels chilly for a moment, gets a little shiver, turns horribly hot and then breaks out into a definite sweat. As a rule, the sweat in *Pyrogenium* is definitely offensive.

Always, in influenza, they complain of intense, generalised aching pains; they ache from head to foot, and are very uncomfortable with it; they are sensitive to pressure, and often move restlessly about in order to ease the painful part.

They suffer from very violent congestive headaches; either severe occipital headaches or, much more commonly, intense throbbing headaches in the temples with a sensation of heat and pressure in the head and often, a damp hot sweat. These congestive headaches are definitely relieved by pressure.

13

A dry mouth is always found in a *Pyrogenium* case, with a good deal of thirst for small quantities of cold water. The tongue tends to become dry, the mouth offensive.

There are two types of tongue in *Pyrogenium* patients. Much the most common is a dry tongue with a somewhat brown coating. Occasionally—less commonly in influenza than in some of their conditions—the tongue has no coating at all; it is deep red and dry, very sensitive, painful and hot, and it tends to crack. This tongue is found more in the frankly septic fevers of *Pyrogenium* than in the catarrhal influenzal states.

These patients tend to have very violent attacks of sneezing, which are brought on by any cold draught. Uncovering them for examination is enough to start them sneezing; sometimes they actually sneeze if they put a hand out of bed—it is cold that always sets them going.

As a rule, the nasal discharge in *Pyrogenium* is thick and gluey, which is difficult to expel. Patients complain that first one side of the nose and then the other gets blocked up; they have great difficulty in clearing it. The right side is blocked more commonly than the left, but it does tend to alternate.

The typical appearance of the *Pyrogenium* throat is relaxed and unhealthy-looking, probably with a certain amount of superficial ulceration of the tonsils and a good deal of offensive gluey postnasal discharge.

In *Pyrogenium* influenzas there is liable to be involvement of the larynx, with a feeling of intense rawness and burning, and an accumulation of the same kind of glairy, sticky mucus which they have difficulty in expelling. There is a very troublesome cough and a good deal of mucus to clear away; the patients cough up sticky, yellowish-coloured mucus.

Most *Pyrogenium* influenza patients have intense ringing in the ears, with a feeling of obstruction, marked tenderness behind the ears, and a severe pressing sensation as if the ears were going to burst. The right ear is much more commonly affected than the left.

Associated with the ear condition is a very similar sensation in the accessory nasal cavities. There is a feeling that the frontal sinuses are blocked, and an intense pressing pain just above the eyes —more commonly above the right eye.

There is also likely to be a similar sensation in the upper jaw from involvement of the antrum, with again the same pressing pain. The antrum pains are liable to go from one side to the other, or to spread right across.

While the condition is acute, the pains are very much aggravated by cold or any active movement of the patient. Coughing, too, increases the pains; the forehead feels as though it would burst, and there is often intense throbbing in the affected area.

14

There is liable to be an extension further back in the accessory sinuses, very often accompanied by an intense pressing pain deep in the skull. It would seem to be an involvement of the sphenoidal cells. The patients very often complain, at this time, of very severe, distressing headache.

These patients have a certain amount of pain and tenderness in the eyes, very often tenderness on pressure. It is usually accompanied by acute photophobia. In fact, there is often photophobia without any acute inflammatory condition in the eyes: the patient seems to be disturbed by light quite apart from the local condition. As a rule the eyes are gummy and sticky rather than showing profuse lachrymation.

Pyrogenium patients always complain of an unpleasant taste—just a feeling of flatness or lack of taste, or a definite putrid taste. They very often say that a lot of stuff accumulates at the back of their throats and, when they spit it out, it has a foul taste. This gives them complete aversion to food, they have no appetite at all. And their very painful throat makes it difficult for them to swallow.

Pyrogenium influenza patients are liable to acute digestive disturbances—enteritis rather than gastritis. They have quite acute abdominal pains accompanied by very violent diarrhœa, always a very offensive and rather profuse watery stool.

Useful for diagnosis is the point that this stinking profuse diarrhœa is not accompanied by a great deal of urging; there is no marked degree of tenesmus. But there is marked abdominal pain, very often in the cæcal region, on the right side of the abdomen, and the pain is very much aggravated by motion. The abdomen is sensitive to touch and the patient rather more comfortable lying on the right side.

There are two other indications for *Pyrogenium* that should be mentioned. Firstly, before the patients develop any signs of cold at all, they are conscious of extreme pains starting in the legs and spreading gradually upwards. Secondly, there is always a marked discrepancy between the pulse rate and the temperature of a *Pyrogenium* patient.

The discrepancy can go either way: rapid pulse and comparatively low temperature or high temperature and comparatively slow pulse.

The typical *Pyrogenium* influenza is quite a serious case. However, the patients do respond astonishingly quickly.

MERCURIUS SOLUBILIS

THE appearance of the typical *Mercurius* influenza is much the same as in *Pyrogenium*, though the patient looks a little more puffy. There may be a localised hectic flush, but it is more common to see a generalised flush in *Mercurius*, often with the face bright red. And there is a damp sweat—peculiarly oily-looking, so that the patient looks greasy.

15

In contrast to the loquacity of *Pyrogenium*, *Mercurius* patients tend to be hurried; their speech is hurried and they rather tumble over their words. There is much more anxiety and restlessness.

Pyrogenium patients, although very ill, are singularly unworried about it. *Mercurius* patients, however, are usually extremely distressed, restless and anxious. Very often, they are definitely depressed, in a *Pulsatilla* way—they weep when shown kindness. Linked with the hurried outlook is a tendency to impatience and irritability.

Their general temperature reaction is another distinguishing point. *Mercurius* patients feel just about as hot as *Pyrogenium* cases, they have the same sort of hot sweat, and are uncomfortable if covered too much and chilly if they uncover; but, there is never the same intense sensitiveness to cold as in *Pyrogenium*—the state is one of alternating between too hot and too cold. If a *Mercurius* patient is kept in a still atmosphere at a moderate temperature, he is fairly comfortable.

Mercurius patients, unlike *Pyrogenium*, have a very marked nightly aggravation; they are very uncomfortable all night, liable to have a marked rise of temperature and apt to sweat more, which only increases their discomfort.

It is difficult to distinguish between the headaches of *Pyrogenium* and *Mercurius* patients. Both suffer from exactly the same type of pressing headache, in just the same situations; both have the same feeling of heat in the head; both seem to get involvement of the frontal sinuses, antrum and ear; and the symptoms are very similar.

Possibly, *Mercurius* patients are a little more sensitive to draughts on the painful areas. More helpfully, they find rather more relief from firm pressure over the painful area than do *Pyrogenium* cases.

As far as thirst is concerned, there is little to distinguish between the two drugs; both are thirsty and want cold drinks. But the actual state of the mouth gives definite indications. The *Mercurius* mouth always shows a swollen, flabby, palish, coated tongue, with a nasty, greasy feel about it, and there is always troublesome, sticky, fairly profuse salivation. (Cf. the dry, brownish tongue of *Pyrogenium*.)

The *Mercurius* tongue is tremulous; it shows a definite fine tremor when protruded. The excessive salivation makes their tongues sticky and they find it difficult to speak and articulate.

The *Mercurius* throat is acutely inflamed, and there is early marked enlargement of the submaxillary glands. The throat itself is very much swollen, dusky, dark red, very tender; it feels hot and burning. The whole of the tissues round the back of the throat seem to be inflamed, and any movement hurts; swallowing is very difficult and may cause stabbing pains that spread out into the ears.

16

The same feeling of soreness and burning extends down the throat, involving the larynx, trachea and bronchi. Any cough is extremely painful; the whole centre of the chest feels raw and as though the mucous membrane had been stripped. The intense inflammation causes hoarseness and, very often, complete loss of voice.

Mercurius influenza patients always have an intense conjunctivitis, with profuse lachrymation of hot, burning tears which seem to excoriate the cheeks. They have severe photophobia, and are peculiarly sensitive to radiant heat—the heat of the fire—which makes their eyes smart and burn.

These patients have a profuse nasal discharge, acrid and watery, which tends to excoriate the upper lip. With it there is intense burning pain in the nose and very violent attacks of sneezing. These attacks will be induced either by going into the open air or coming into a warm room—either heat or cold will set them going—and any draught is liable to precipitate a violent bout of sneezing.

There is a tendency for the watery discharge to become thicker, and greenish in colour. It is then that the patients are liable to have intense pains radiating out into the antrum, underneath the eyes or up into the frontal sinuses.

With the intensely inflamed throat of *Mercurius* influenzas there is liable to be pretty acute involvement of the middle ear. It usually starts with a feeling that the ears are choked and stopped-up; and there may be a certain amount of buzzing in the ears. Very quickly the ear becomes painful. There is a feeling of increased tension and the ear throbs

Pain tends to spread right up the side of the head and, very often, involves half the head. There is marked tenderness of the mastoid region, very often enlargement of the post auricular glands, spreading down into the neck; extremely injected drums and early rupture.

Mercurius patients have complete loss of appetite in influenza. With their acutely inflamed throats they can hardly swallow. Moreover, there is constant accumulation of unpleasant saliva, the swallowing of which is both painful and also liable to cause a feeling of intense nausea.

These patients have generalised muscular pains. They feel stiffness in the back of the neck, down the back, in their arms and legs; and it is painful to move.

And, not only the tongue but the whole patient becomes tremulous in a *Mercurius* influenza. Hands become shaky and all fine movements tremulous.

KALIUM BICHROMICUM

KALI BIC. is worthy of mention because of its affinity to accessory sinuses.

The typical *Kali bic.* influenza patient is rather pale, with red blotches about the face.

Discharges are irritating, and the upper lip swollen and reddish, due to coryza.

The mental state of typical *Kali bic.* influenza patients is one of mild discouragement. They have difficulty in thinking, any attempt at mental effort is almost impossible, and they are rather discouraged and hopeless. They feel very weak, tired and weary, and like to be left in peace.

Kali bic. influenzas are generally definitely chilly.

The patients have a good deal of generalised, wandering rheumatic pains—the wandering character is important—first in the shoulder, then in the elbow, the back or the knee, and so on. These pains grow worse if the patients are cold; in bed, with plenty of hot-water bottles, they are fairly comfortable.

A characteristic of *Kali bic.* influenza is the patients' really bad period in the morning. They have a temperature aggravation about 2 or 3 in the morning. Their real discomfort, however, is between 6 a.m. and 8 a.m.—very much later than one would expect from a *Kali* salt.

There is a very copious nasal discharge which feels hot and burning. It is usually white, or slightly yellow, in colour; rather stringy, and always accompanied by a feeling of extreme obstruction at the root of the nose. The patient feels as if the root of the nose were completely blocked, swollen, full and hot; he has violent sneezing attacks, with pain spreading out from the root of the nose to the external angle of the eye.

The same blockage occurs in the frontal sinuses or antrum, again with the feeling of tension. The headache, or face pain, is very much aggravated by movement, but definitely relieved by pressure. It usually tends to be confined to one side.

When the pain becomes intense, it is very liable to produce a sensation of nausea and may actually make the patient sick. It is definitely relieved by hot applications and is sensitive to cold.

Occasionally, one meets a case in which the pain is located in one small spot just above one of the frontal sinuses: this is almost diagnostic of *Kali bic*.

As a rule, the mouth is dry; and the tongue has a slight coating, either white or yellowish. There may be a certain amount of ropy saliva, but it is much more likely to be a postnasal discharge and stringy in character.

The throat in *Kali bic.* tends to be very red and swollen, with a very definite œdematous appearance. There may be a very much swollen, œdematous uvula and, almost certainly, signs of acute follicular tonsillitis. The throat is always very painful, and—a *Kali bic.* characteristic—it is very painful for the patient to put out his tongue; the pulling on the muscles at the root of the tongue hurts. Another characteristic is the strange sensation of a hair across the soft palate.

There is very early hoarseness in *Kali bic.* influenzas, with an accumulation of mucus in the larynx. It is the same kind of stringy white, or whitish yellow, mucus and is coughed up with great difficulty.

As a rule, there is a spread downwards from the larynx, with a feeling of great tightness in the chest. Very often, there is accumulation of mucus in the larger bronchi, sometimes spreading into the smaller bronchi, becoming a definite bronchitis and accompanied by wheezing. There is a very violent, difficult cough, and expectoration of large quantities of very stringy, adherent mucus.

Short of that, the accumulation of stuff on the larynx is liable to cause an intensely irritating, tickling sensation which excites a very spasmodic cough, almost like whooping cough.

The patients nearly always say that they are very exhausted by the effort of coughing; they are often sweaty, and get extreme palpitation.

There is some involvement of the ear, with blockage of the Eustachian tube and fullness in the ears; it may develop into a definite middle ear abscess. Where this occurs in *Kali bic.*, there may be extreme swelling of the external ear as well as the involvement of the middle ear.

Most *Kali bic.* influenzas have gastric catarrh. They may have acute gastritis, with troublesome nausea and vomiting of a quantity of unpleasant glairy mucus. This is very difficult to bring up, and the effort of vomiting is apt to produce a most intense headache. The gastric catarrh may spread down and become a duodenal catarrh, with a certain amount of jaundice.

The *Kali bic.* chilliness is rather "different": it is particularly situated in the back of the neck. Patients hate to have their necks uncovered; they are much more comfortable with a hot-water bottle tucked into the nape of their neck. The chilliness sometimes spreads down the back, and they then complain of feeling chilly in the small of their back.

Some *Kali bic.* influenza patients have an astonishing sensitiveness of the hand; they feel as if their hands were bruised. Shaking hands is apt to cause them pain; they describe the same feeling of bruisedness in the soles of their feet if they stand on them.

INDEX TO DRUGS